I0820247

IN-DEMAND CAREERS

BE A NURSE PRACTITIONER

by Marne Ventura

BrightPoint Press

San Diego, CA

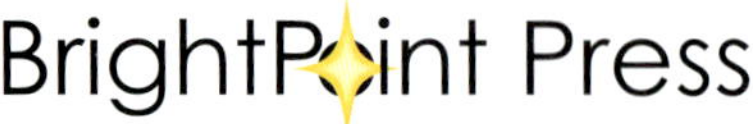

an imprint of ReferencePoint Press, Inc.
Printed in the United States

For more information, contact:
BrightPoint Press
PO Box 27779
San Diego, CA 92198
www.BrightPointPress.com

LIBRARY OF CONGRESS CATALOGING-IN-PUBLICATION DATA

Names: Ventura, Marne author
Title: Be a nurse practitioner / by Marne Ventura.
Description: San Diego, CA: ReferencePoint Press, [2026] | Series: In-demand careers | Includes bibliographical references and index. | Audience term: juvenile | Audience: Grades 7–9 BrightPoint Press
Identifiers: LCCN 2024060066 (print) | LCCN 2024060067 (eBook) | ISBN 9781678211202 hardcover | ISBN 9781678211219 (eBook)
Subjects: LCSH: Nurse practitioners--Juvenile literature | Nursing--Vocational guidance--Juvenile literature | Nursing--Juvenile literature
Classification: LCC RT82.8 .V46 2026 (print) | LCC RT82.8 (eBook) | DDC 610.7306/92--dc23/eng/20250207
LC record available at https://lccn.loc.gov/2024060066
LC eBook record available at https://lccn.loc.gov/2024060067

CONTENTS

AT A GLANCE

- A nurse practitioner (NP) is a registered nurse (RN) with advanced education and experience. NPs perform many of the same duties as doctors.
- NPs do physical exams, diagnose and treat illnesses, and prescribe medicine.
- NPs order tests and analyze test results. They create patient care plans and refer patients to specialists.
- NPs record medical histories and advise patients on how to stay healthy.
- Training to become an NP takes 6 to 8 years. NPs first become RNs. Then they do graduate programs.
- NPs work in doctor's offices, hospitals, emergency rooms, and nursing homes.

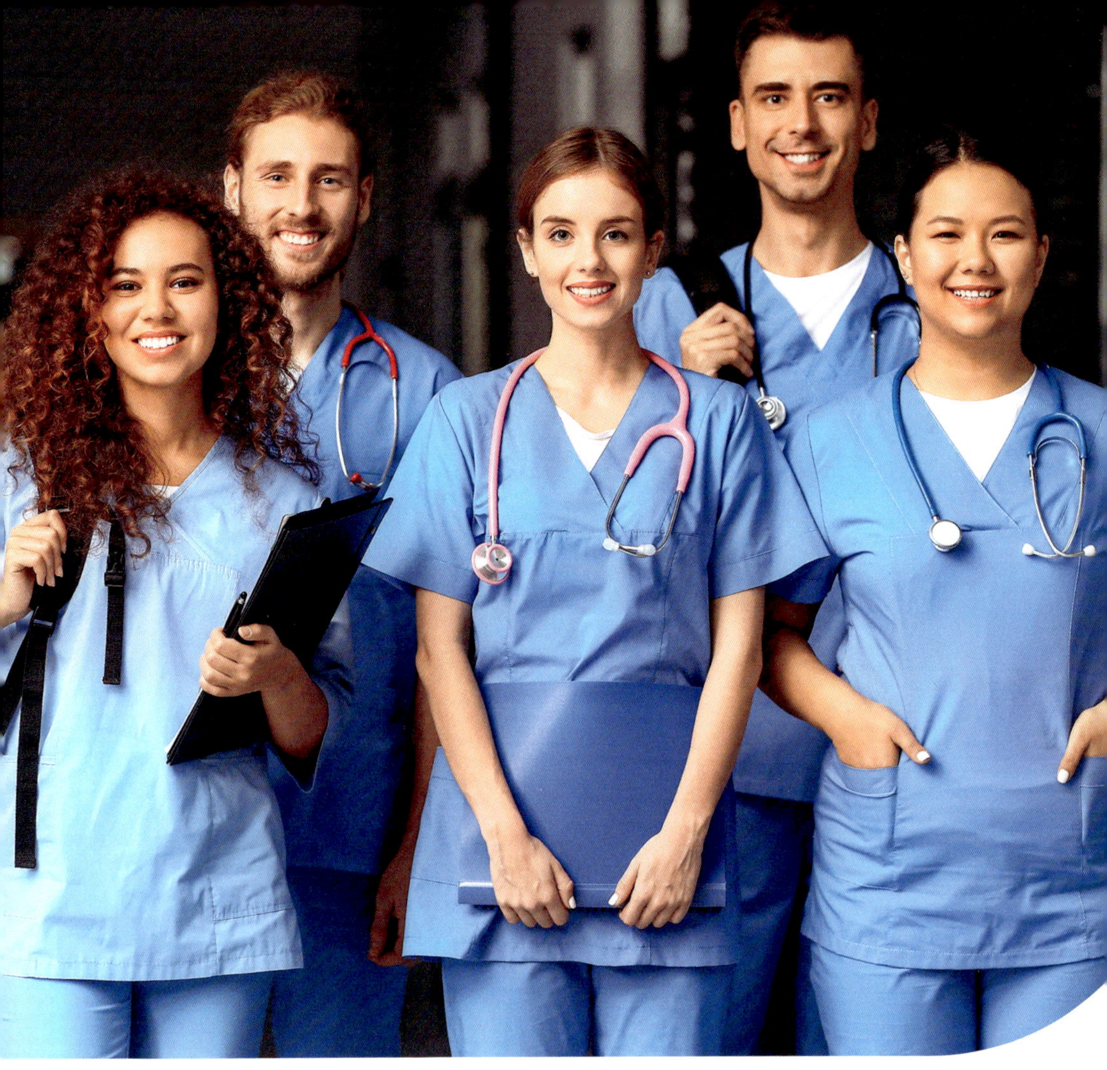

- NPs can specialize in psychiatric care, family practice, internal medicine, pediatric or neonatal care, or women's reproductive health.
- Because of a shortage of doctors and nurses, the demand for NPs will rise during the next 10 years.

UNSUNG HERO

Alison is a nurse practitioner (NP). She works in a clinic. She gives allergy tests. She **diagnoses** patients. She also prescribes allergy medicine.

Julie is one of Alison's patients. Alison gives Julie her weekly allergy shots. Each shot contains a tiny amount of **allergen**. Over time, Julie's body learns not to react to the allergen.

When giving a shot, nurses clean the skin before injecting the needle. This decreases the likelihood of infection.

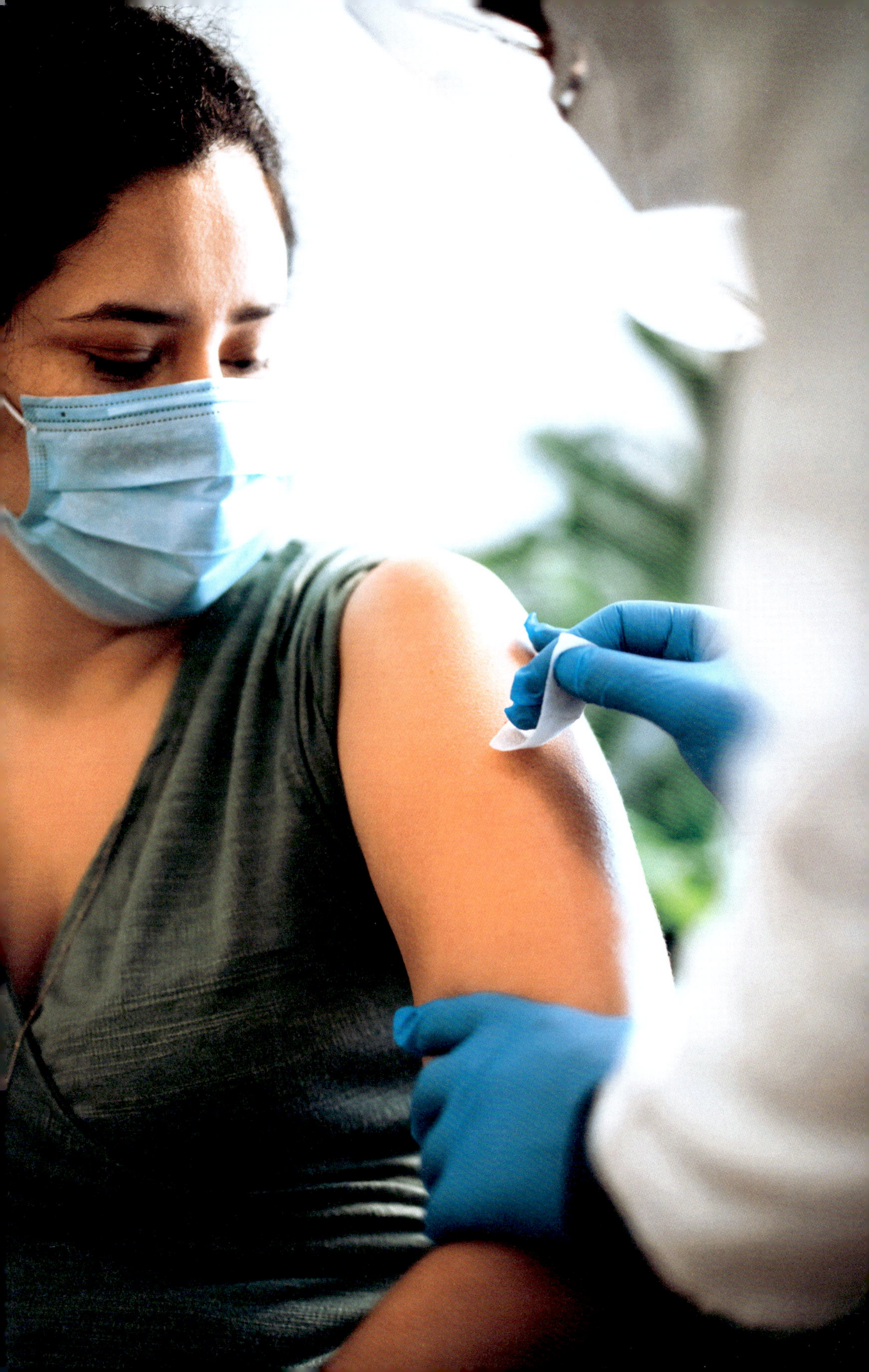

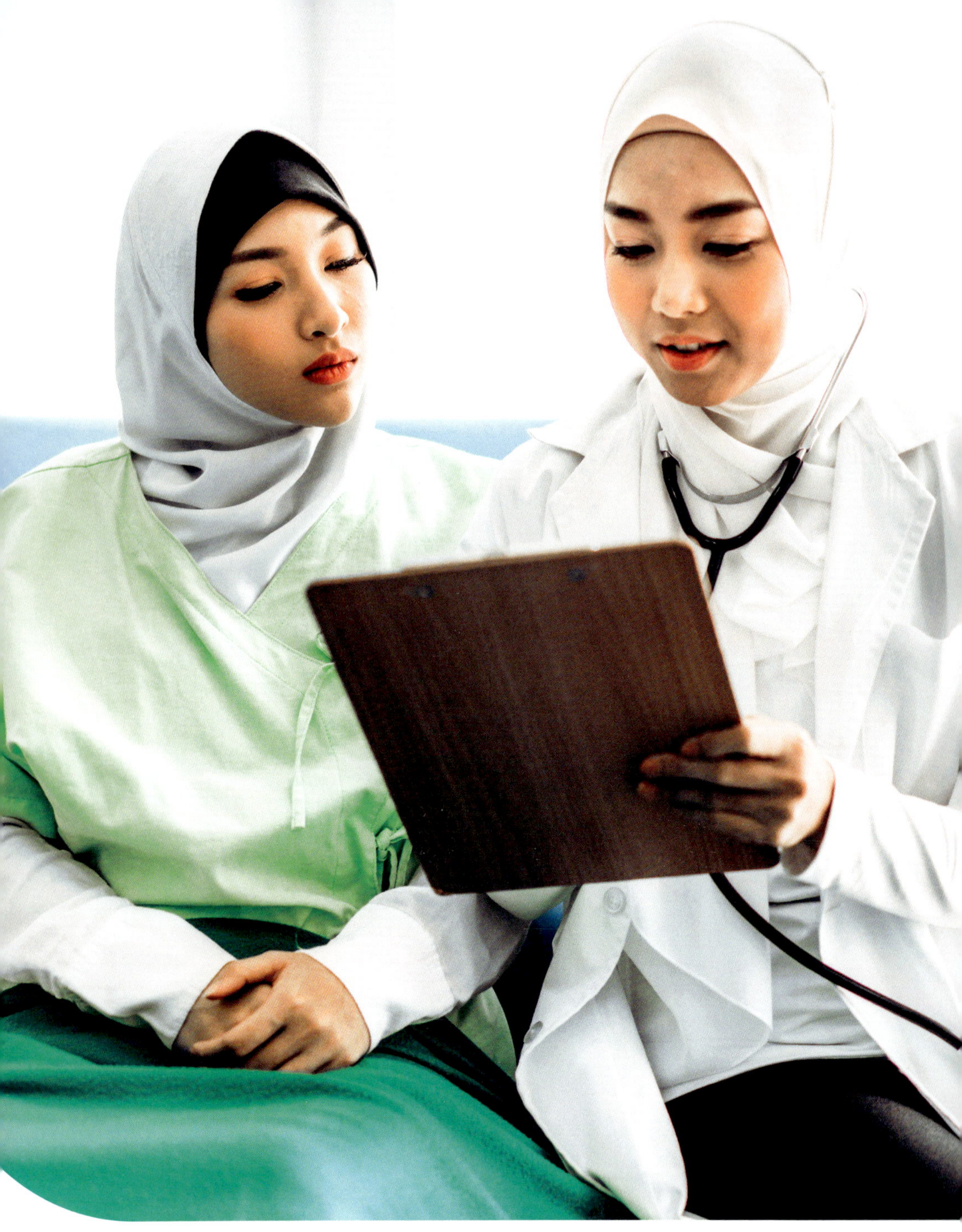

Health care providers check in with patients about their family backgrounds and medical histories. This helps identify any potential issues or allergies to medicine.

At Julie's first visit, Alison notices Julie's cough. She asks her about it. Julie has seen several doctors. They could not find a cause for it. Julie's cough lasts for weeks. Alison knows Julie's cough should have gone away. Instead, it seems to be getting worse.

During Alison's NP training, she learned about a test to check a patient's airway. The airway leads from the throat to the lungs. Alison thinks there is a problem in Julie's airway. She asks Julie if she would be willing to have one of the doctors do the test. Julie agrees.

The doctor finds the problem. Julie has a rare condition. Scar tissue blocks most of her airway. She is breathing through an opening about the width of a drinking straw.

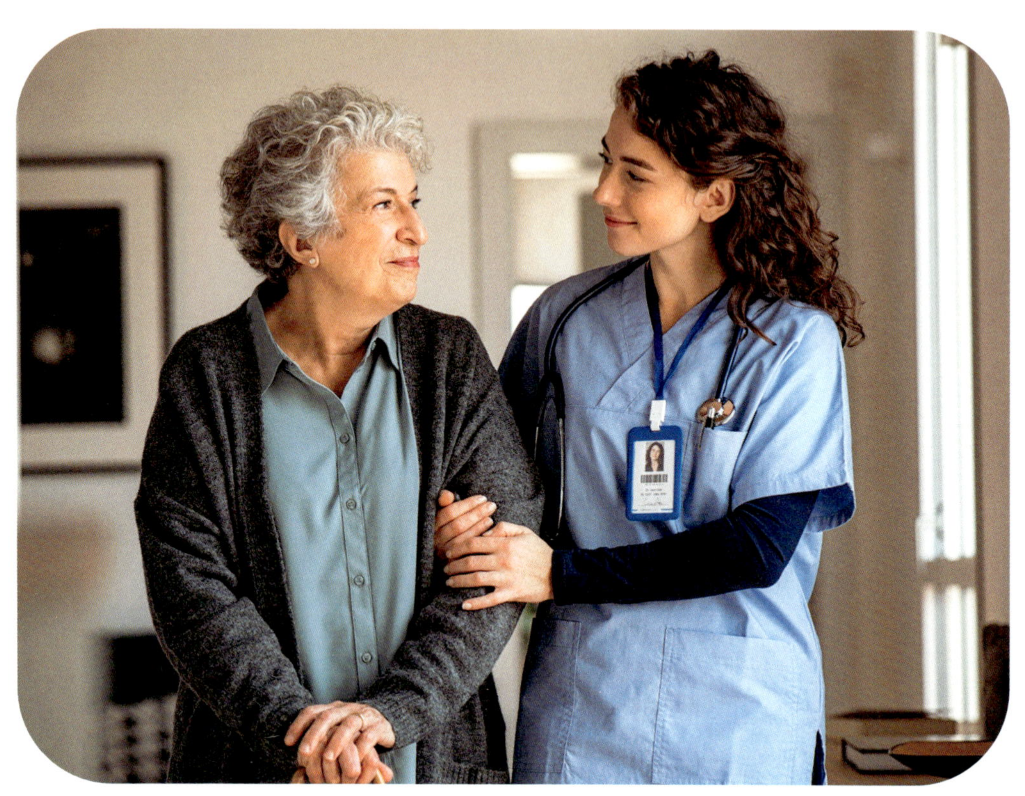

NPs work with many patients. They take care of patients' health care needs.

Julie needs treatment. Without it, her airway might close all the way. She could die.

Julie calls NP Alison her unsung hero. She says, "It was her persistence and diligence and her listening to me and taking me seriously that got my diagnosis in a timely enough fashion to do something about it."[1]

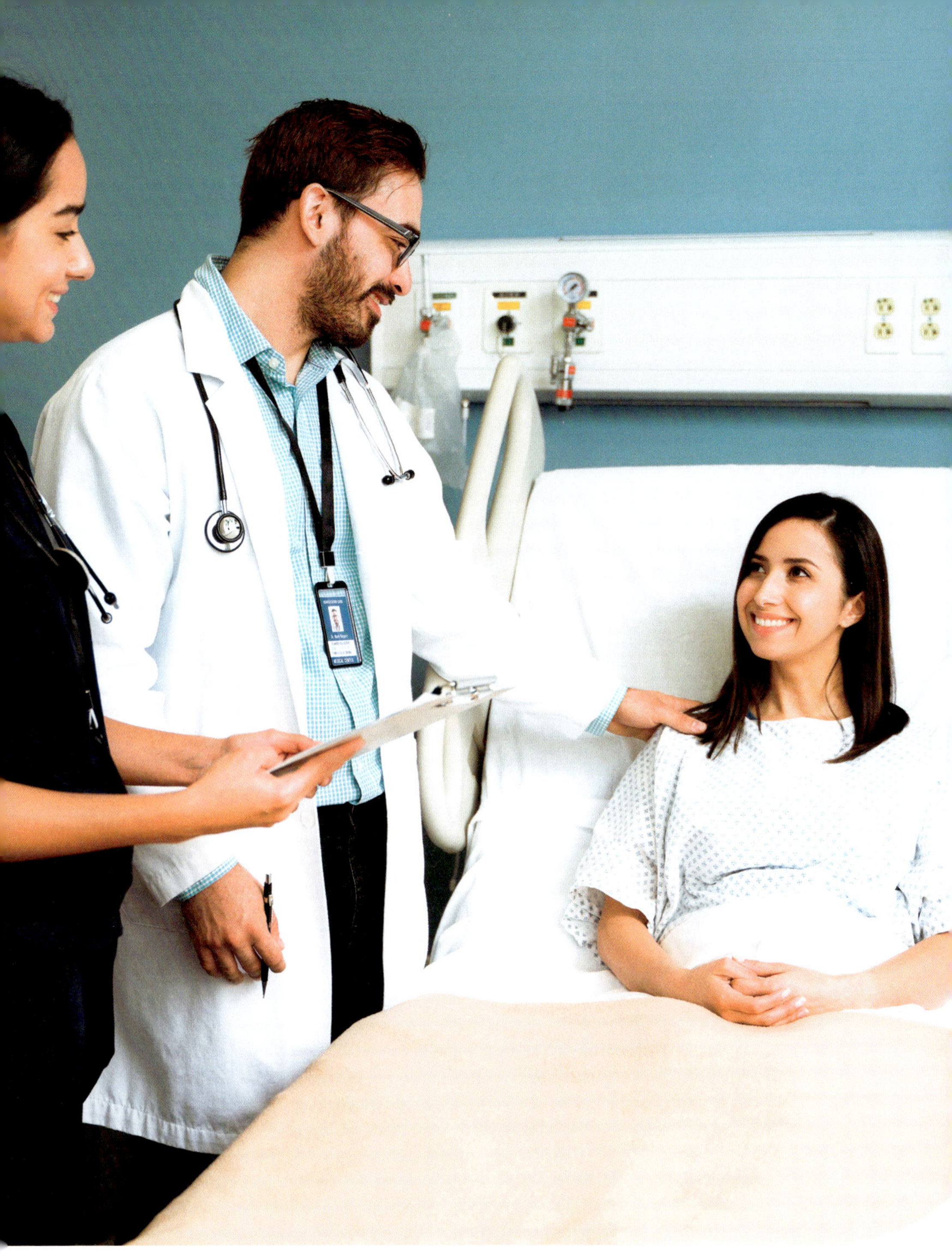

After operations, NPs help patients recover. They come up with care plans.

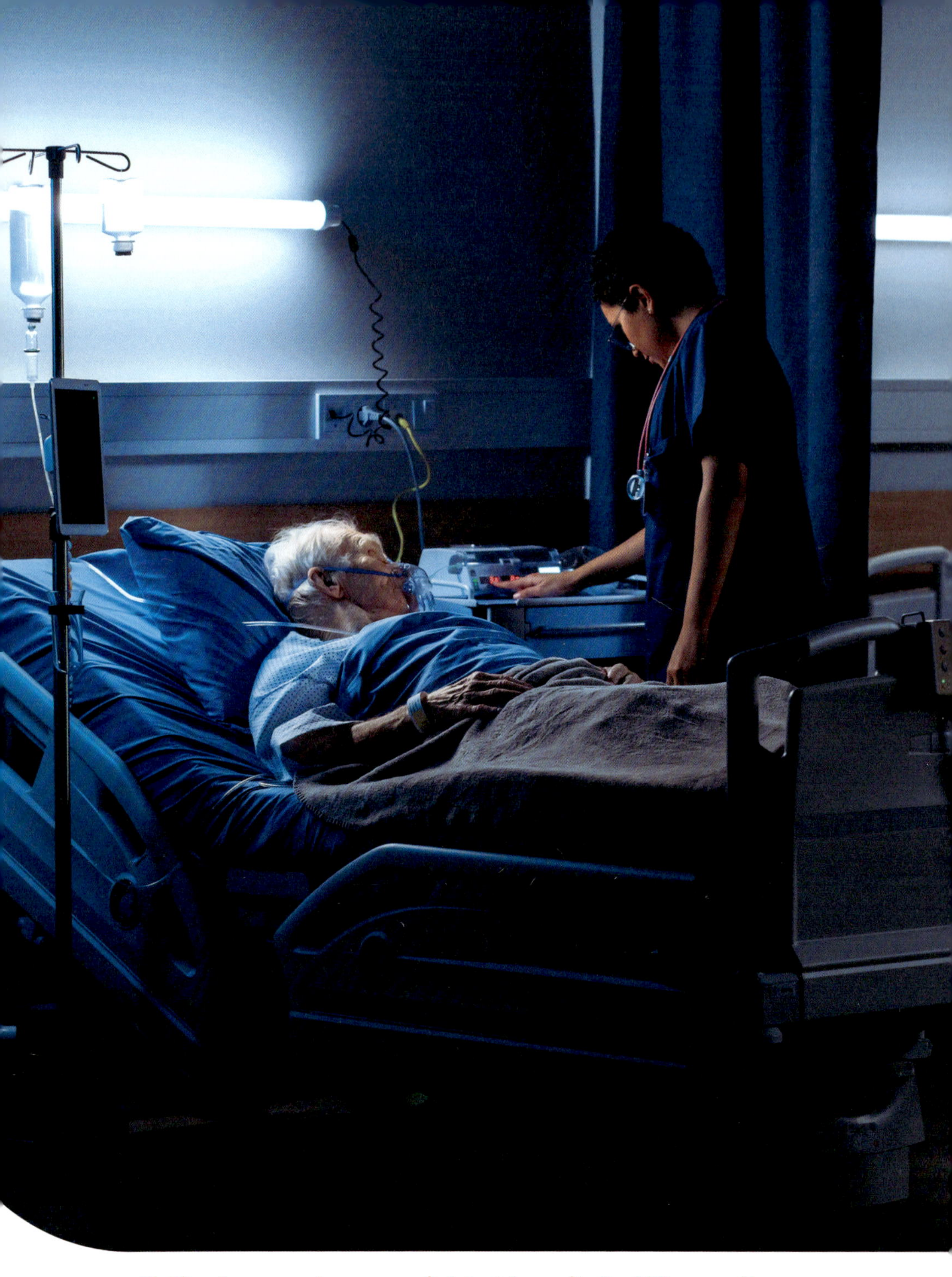

Patients may stay overnight at hospitals. NPs monitor the patients' health while they rest.

WHAT IS A NURSE PRACTITIONER?

NPs like Alison work with patients of all ages. They work in clinics and hospitals. They treat different types of problems. NPs may perform physical exams. They diagnose diseases. They also prescribe medication. These are all things that doctors usually do.

An NP is a registered nurse (RN) with more education. Both an RN and NP earn a 2-year or a 4-year degree. In addition, NPs also earn a graduate degree. They gain more experience and add to their skillsets. Both RNs and NPs care for patients. RNs work under doctors who diagnose and treat patients. NPs can do these tasks without a doctor's supervision.

CHAPTER ONE

WHAT DOES A NURSE PRACTITIONER DO?

NPs care for people of all ages. They help patients stay healthy. They do yearly checkups. They check that their patients' vital organs are working well. They help patients stay up-to-date on vaccines.

NPs also treat patients who are ill or hurt. They ask patients about their symptoms. These are signs of a medical condition. NPs may order and read test results. They make treatment plans. In most states, NPs can

NPs interact with many patients. They learn to pay attention to patients' needs and form positive relationships.

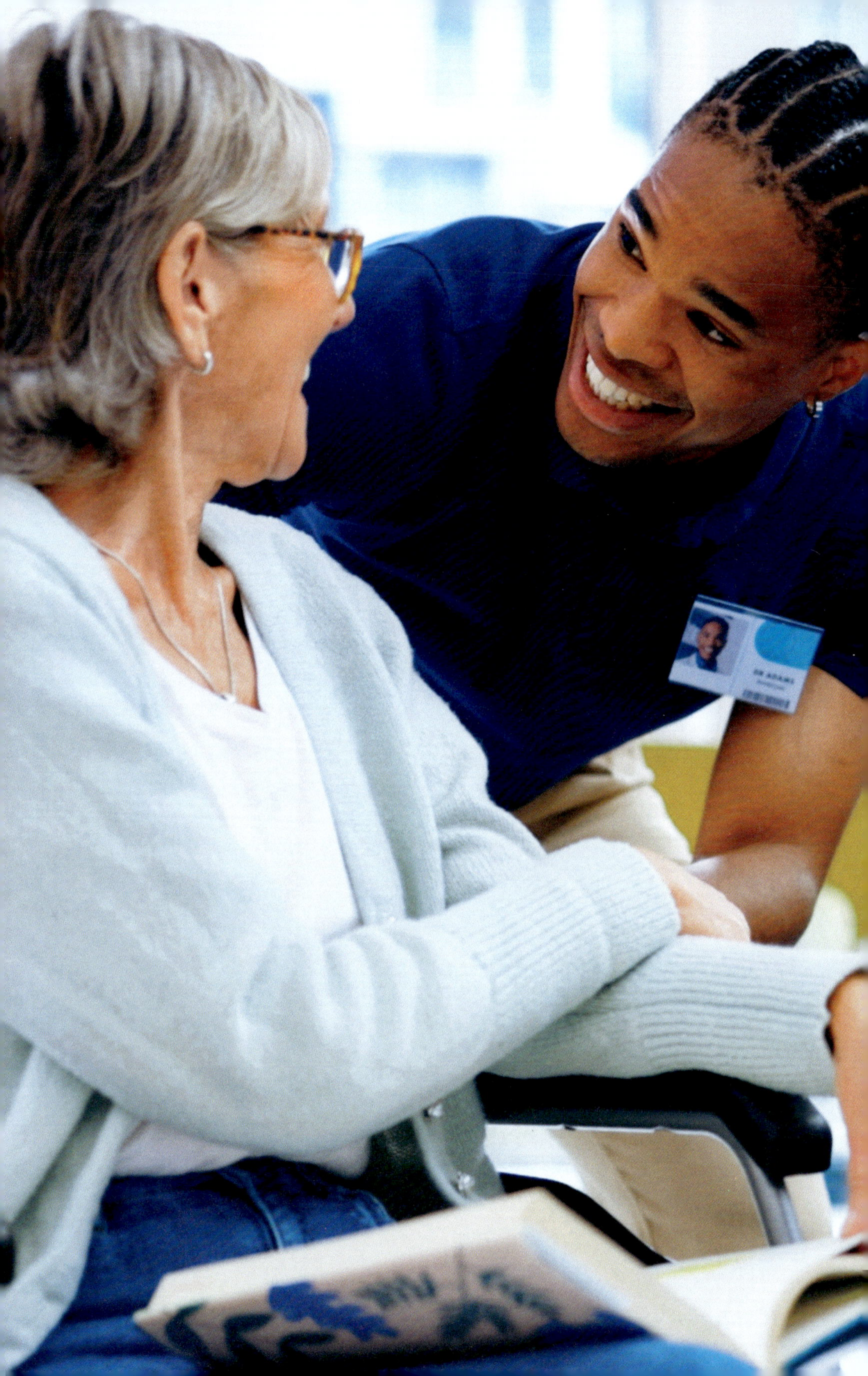

prescribe medicine. This is something that doctors usually do, and that RNs cannot do.

PRIMARY AND ACUTE CARE

Some NPs are primary care providers. This is a doctor or nurse whom a patient sees for yearly checkups. Patients may see them when they feel unwell or have a minor injury. The University of California at Davis Health Blog defines their role. It says,

> *A primary care provider may also be thought of as a "general practitioner," or your personal doctor. They are . . . a "health care home base" for your overall wellness. [They] also give referrals to specialists when you need additional medical expertise to treat a specific condition.*[2]

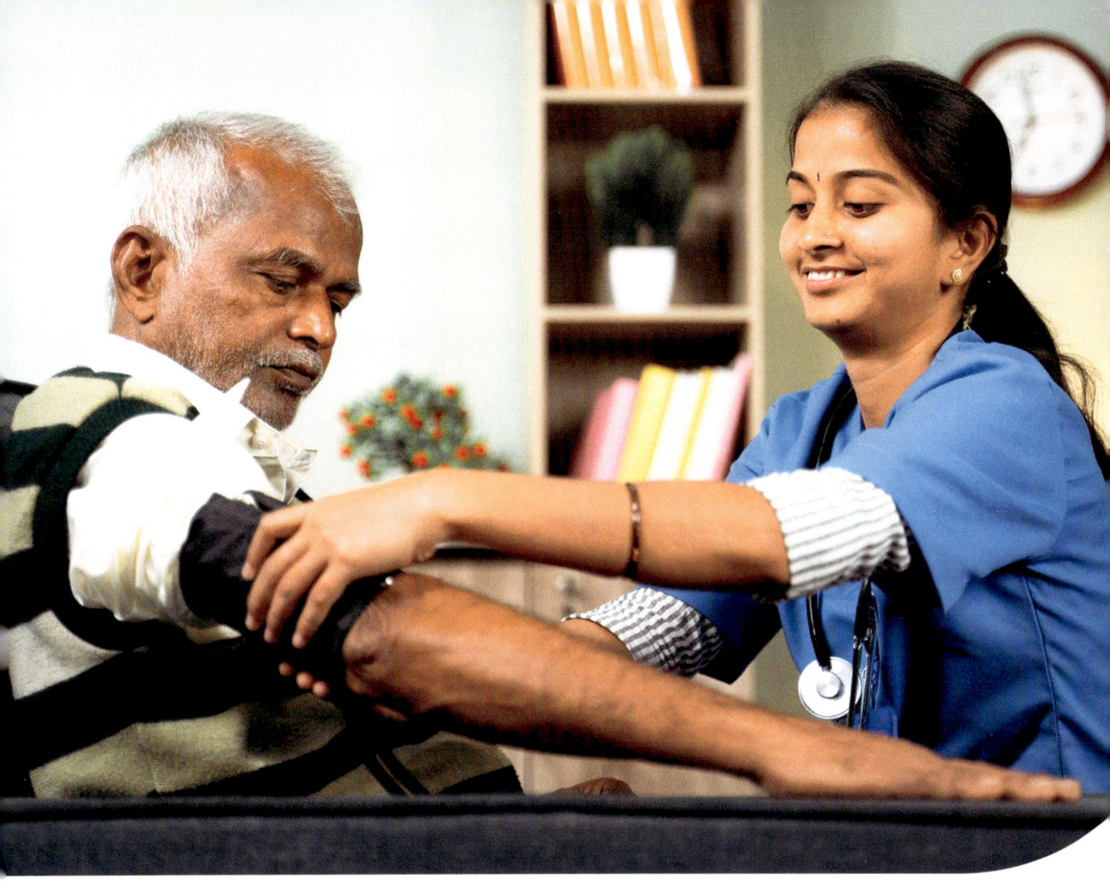

NPs may check blood pressure during checkups.

NPs provide different types of primary care. Primary care NPs see patients for annual checkups. They help prevent illnesses. They also help treat **chronic conditions**. Primary care programs include family practice and adult care.

Acute care NPs support patients when they suddenly become ill. Most acute care NPs work in hospitals. They care for patients in intensive care units (ICUs). This is where seriously ill patients are cared for. NPs may also work in hospital emergency rooms (ERs). Acute care NPs clean and dress wounds. They insert intravenous (IV) lines. This gives patients medicine through their veins. NPs give blood **transfusions**. They use medical equipment such as ventilators. This is a machine that helps a person breathe. Acute care includes pediatrics, psychiatric-mental health, women's health, and neonatal care.

NP SPECIALTIES

NPs working in primary and acute care can have different specialties. Some work with patients in a certain age group. Family NPs see patients of all ages. Neonatal NPs treat newborns. They monitor infants with low birth weights, heart problems, or illnesses. They provide support to the families of these infants. They use medical equipment such as breathing or feeding tubes to help infants perform these functions.

Pediatric NPs provide care for babies, children, and teens.

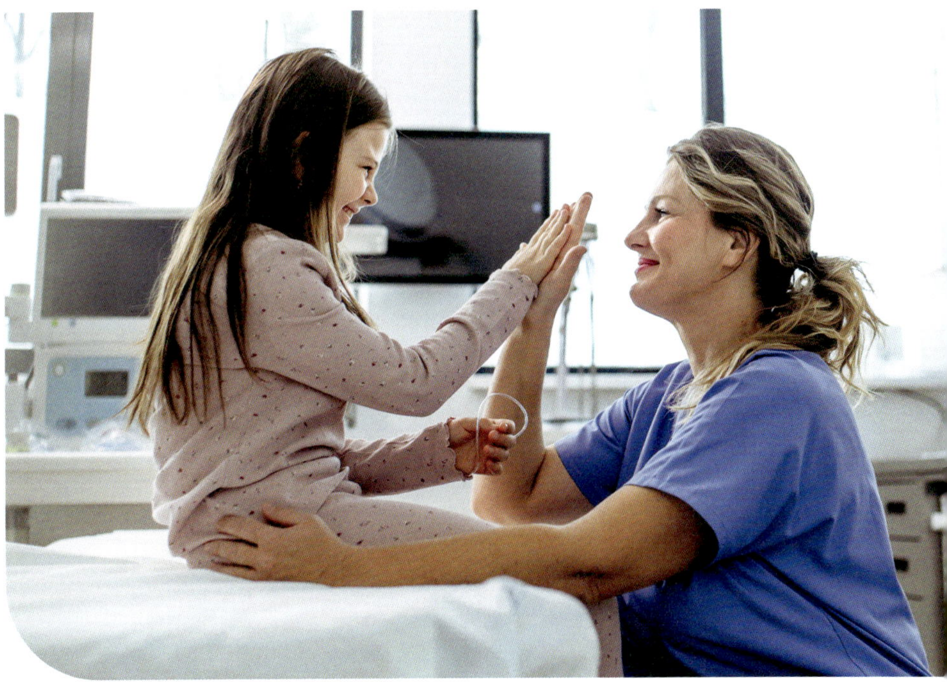

Gerontology NPs care for older adults. They work in hospitals, long-term care homes, and private homes. They do routine health checks to help patients manage diseases such as **diabetes**. They also help patients recover from injuries. This includes falls or strokes. A stroke is caused by a blood clot or burst blood vessel in the brain.

Some NPs work with internal medicine doctors. These doctors specialize in parts of the body. This includes the heart

Popular NP Specialties

Family practice is the most common NP specialty. About 70 percent of NPs work in this field. It is the most popular NP job. The second most in-demand specialty is adult-gerontology primary care. The third is mental health.

or stomach. Obstetrics and gynecology (OB-GYN) NPs provide **reproductive health care** for women.

NPs also specialize based on illnesses. Oncology NPs care for cancer patients. They help patients manage pain. They oversee transfusions. A psychiatric NP cares for patients with mental illness. Some patients have depression or anxiety. Others may have eating disorders or behavior problems. Psychiatric NPs examine, test, and diagnose patients. They may design treatment plans. A treatment plan might include prescribing the right medication. It might include counseling. NPs help patients by asking questions about their well-being. They show care and compassion when listening to a patient's needs.

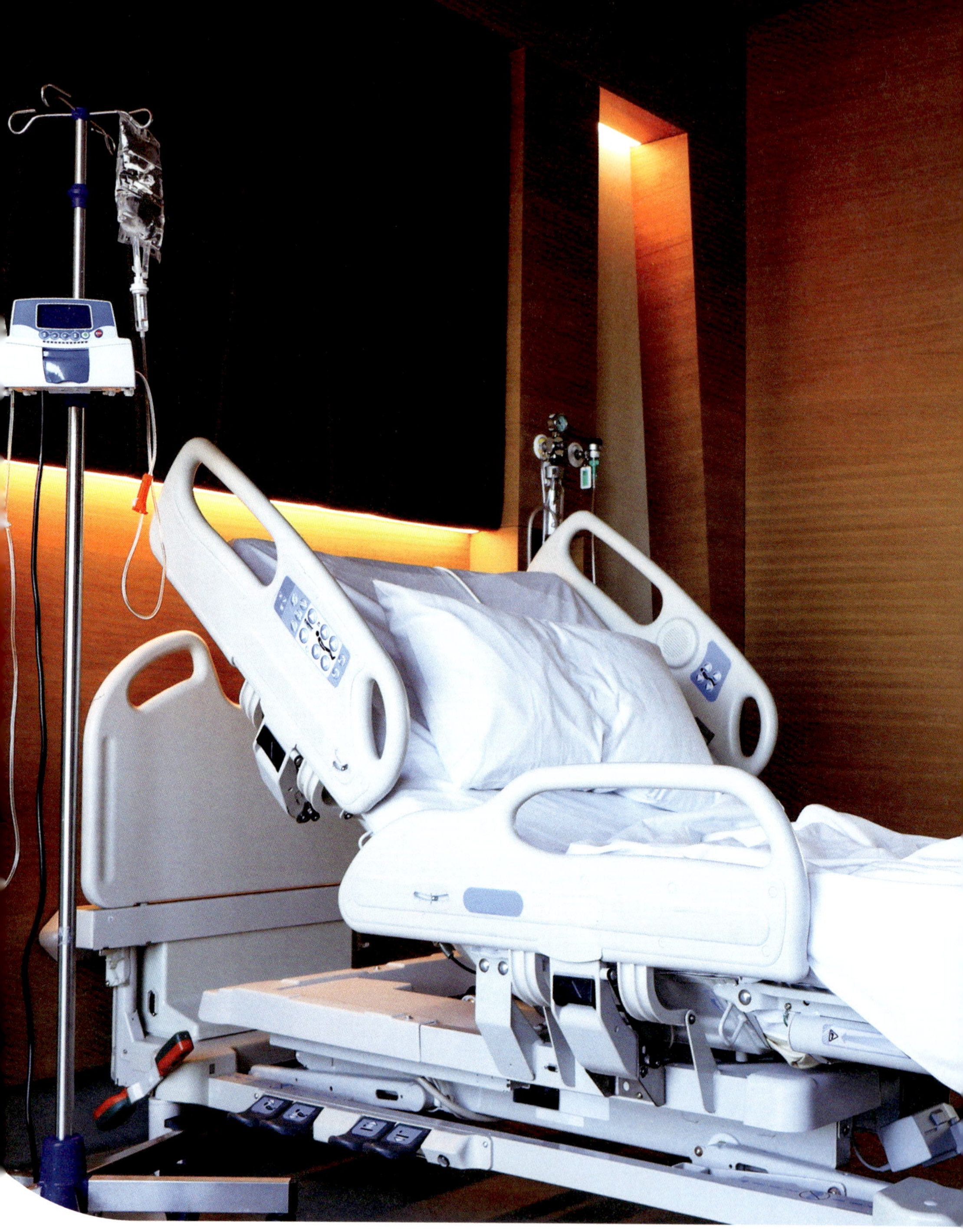

Hospital rooms are equipped with electronic beds that make it easier for caregivers to move patients and keep them comfortable.

Depending on their specialty, NPs can work in clinics, hospitals, or homes. Primary care NPs often work in doctor's offices. Their daily schedule is usually 8:00 a.m. to 5:00 p.m., Monday through Friday. Acute care NPs work in ERs or hospitals. They might work nights and weekends. NPs may be on call. This means they are required to come to work right away if called, even outside of their working schedules.

According to the University of Tulsa, "Understanding the distinctions between these roles [primary care vs. acute care] can help nurses determine which specialty is the ideal fit for them."[3]

CHAPTER TWO

BECOMING A NURSE PRACTITIONER

The first step to becoming an NP is to become an RN. Some RNs may first complete an associate degree in nursing (ADN). It is a program that takes 2 years. Some RNs go directly to a 4-year degree. They earn a bachelor of science in nursing (BSN). RNs with 4-year degrees and clinical practice are ready for graduate school. ADNs and BSNs programs are offered at many public and private colleges.

Nursing programs include lectures, labs, and clinical work.

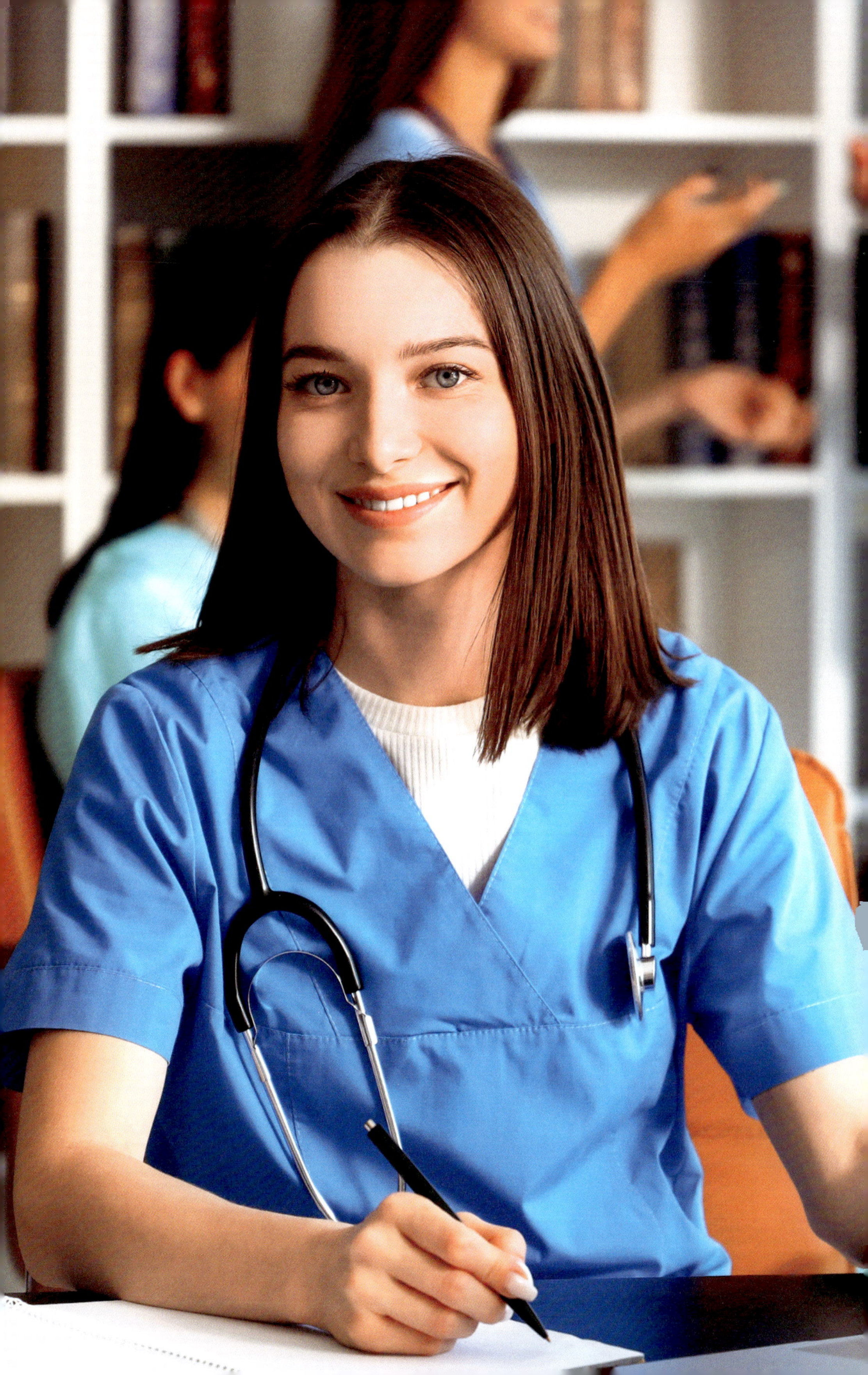

RN students take life science classes. These classes include biology and chemistry. RNs also take math, psychology, and sociology. Psychology helps RNs understand how the brain works. Sociology helps RNs learn about social factors that affect patient well-being and health.

Nursing students go through school together. They share knowledge and support each other.

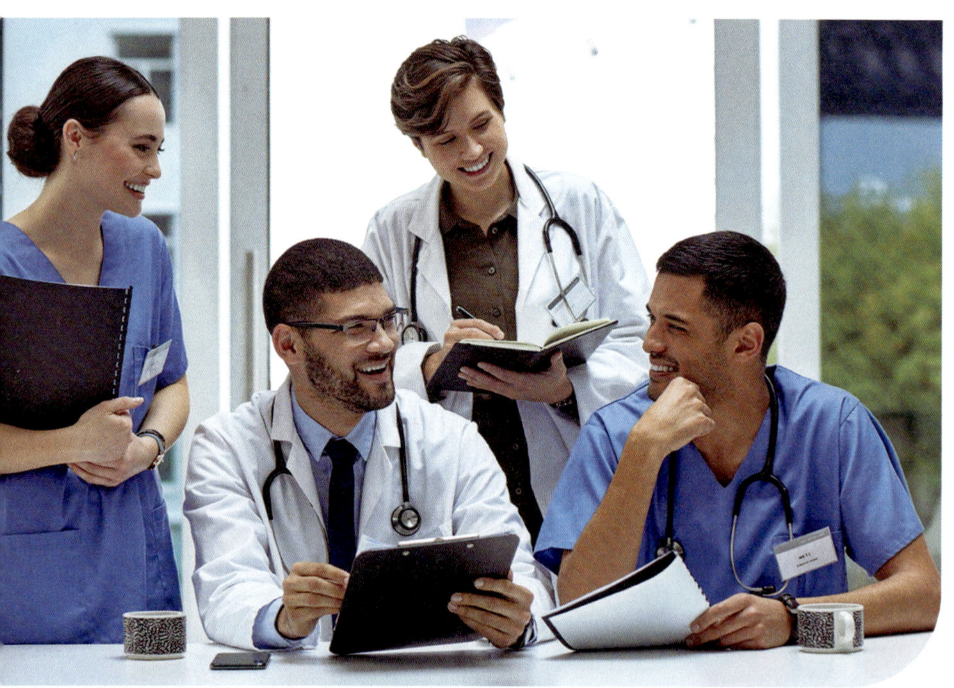

Students learn the basics of patient care. They practice working with patients. RNs in clinics or hospitals help them learn. First, students observe. Then they learn how to give medicine. They may order, give, and read test results. They also learn different ways to communicate with patients. They give both verbal and written directions.

LICENSING AND EXPERIENCE

After completing a college program, each graduate must pass a test. It is called the National Council Licensure Examination for Registered Nurses (NCLEX-RN). The questions are mostly multiple-choice. The test questions ask how to care for patients. They may also ask ways to promote patients' mental and social health.

The final step is to get a license from the Board of Nursing. Requirements vary by state. Students must pass a background check. Often, they must get fingerprinted as well. The National Council of State Boards of Nursing (NCSBN) requires certain hours spent practicing. They check the number of hours a student has worked with patients. Clinical practice hour requirements vary. Some states may require 250 hours. Others may require more than 1,000 hours.

Many future NPs can choose to work for a few years as RNs. Some NP graduate programs require 1 to 2 years of RN experience. RNs might work in hospital ERs. Some work at family practice clinics. RNs might work in neonatal ICUs or OB-GYN offices. On-the-job learning helps

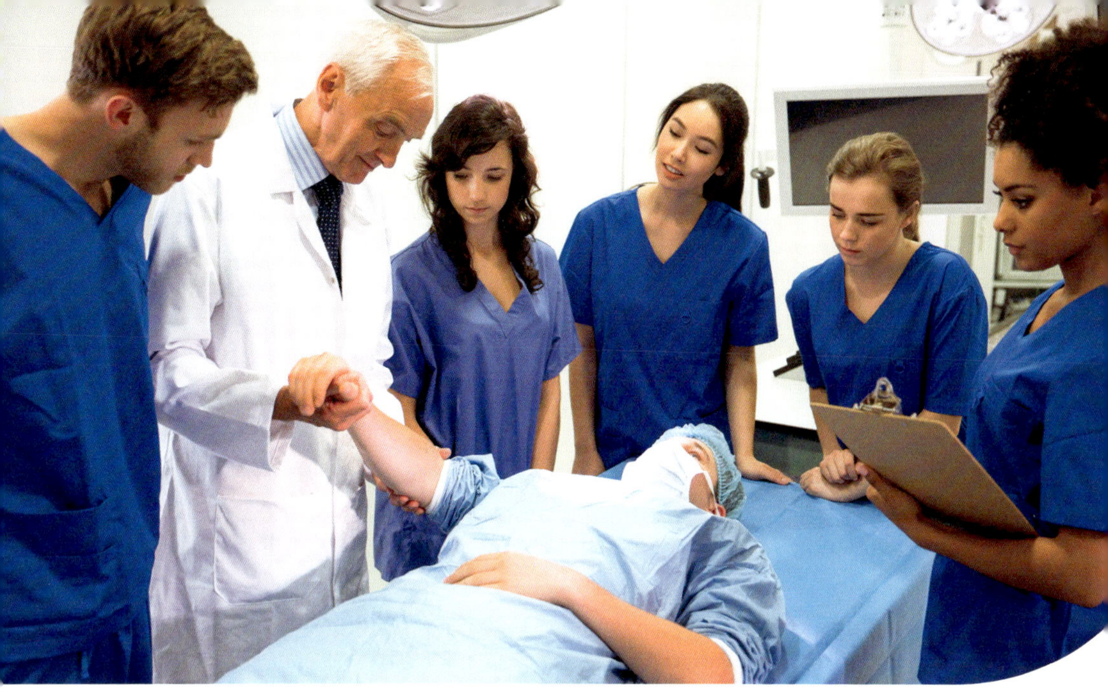

Working with manikins helps nursing students practice clinical skills such as taking vital signs.

RNs improve their caregiving skills. These experiences also help nurses decide what kind of care they prefer to give.

GRADUATE DEGREE PROGRAMS

NPs need to earn their master of science in nursing (MSN). They can also earn their doctor of nursing practice (DNP). MSN programs take anywhere from 18 months to 3 years to complete. DNP programs might take 3 to 4 years. When completed, students must get certified. This happens by their state Board of Nursing.

NP programs focus on a student's chosen specialty. NPs can choose a sub-specialty as well. These usually require a certificate. Some NPs may be trained in a specialty by the doctor they work with.

Doctor of Nursing Practice (DNP)

A doctor of nursing practice (DNP) program is the highest degree an NP can have. It prepares RNs for leadership roles. They can have more influence over health care policies. DNPs can earn more money, too. DNPs can be head nurses, nurse educators, and college professors. They can also be CEOs of health care organizations. This degree is not needed to be an NP.

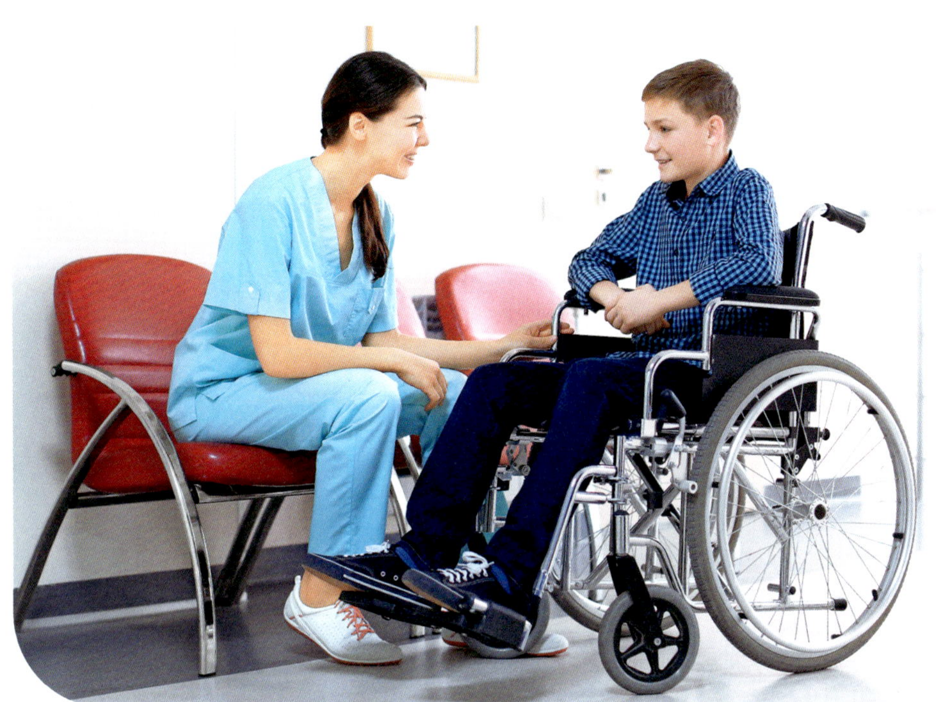

Orthopedic NPs help treat musculoskeletal conditions such as broken bones.

These specialties include occupational health NPs. They treat patients with workplace injuries. Cardiology NPs care for patients with heart disease. Aesthetics NPs do cosmetic procedures in spas. Hospice NPs work with end-of-life patients.

Future NPs go to a graduate degree program in their chosen specialty. To apply, RNs submit past documents. These include courses and grades earned from their BSN program. They also submit their RN license. Most schools ask for personal essays. Applicants describe why they want to become NPs. They may also need recommendation letters. These are letters from past professors or work supervisors that help explain why applicants are good fits. Testing is also required for some graduate programs. The Graduate Records Exam (GRE) is a multiple-choice test. It measures reading, writing, and thinking skills. The Medical College Admission Test (MCAT) is another exam. It tests knowledge and skills needed to provide quality health care.

It takes a lot of time and hard work to become an NP but the profession offers

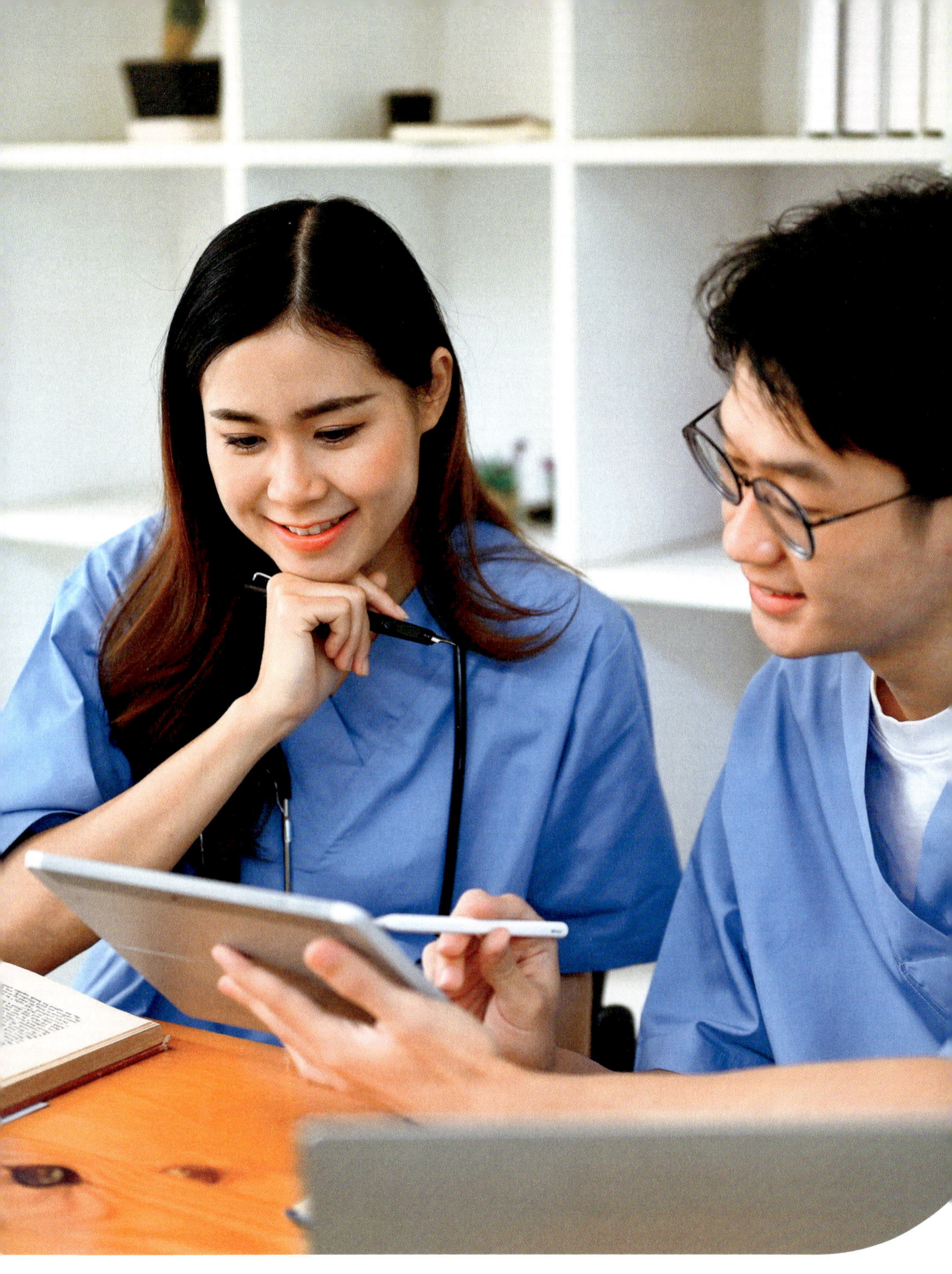

Tutors can help nursing students study for important tests.

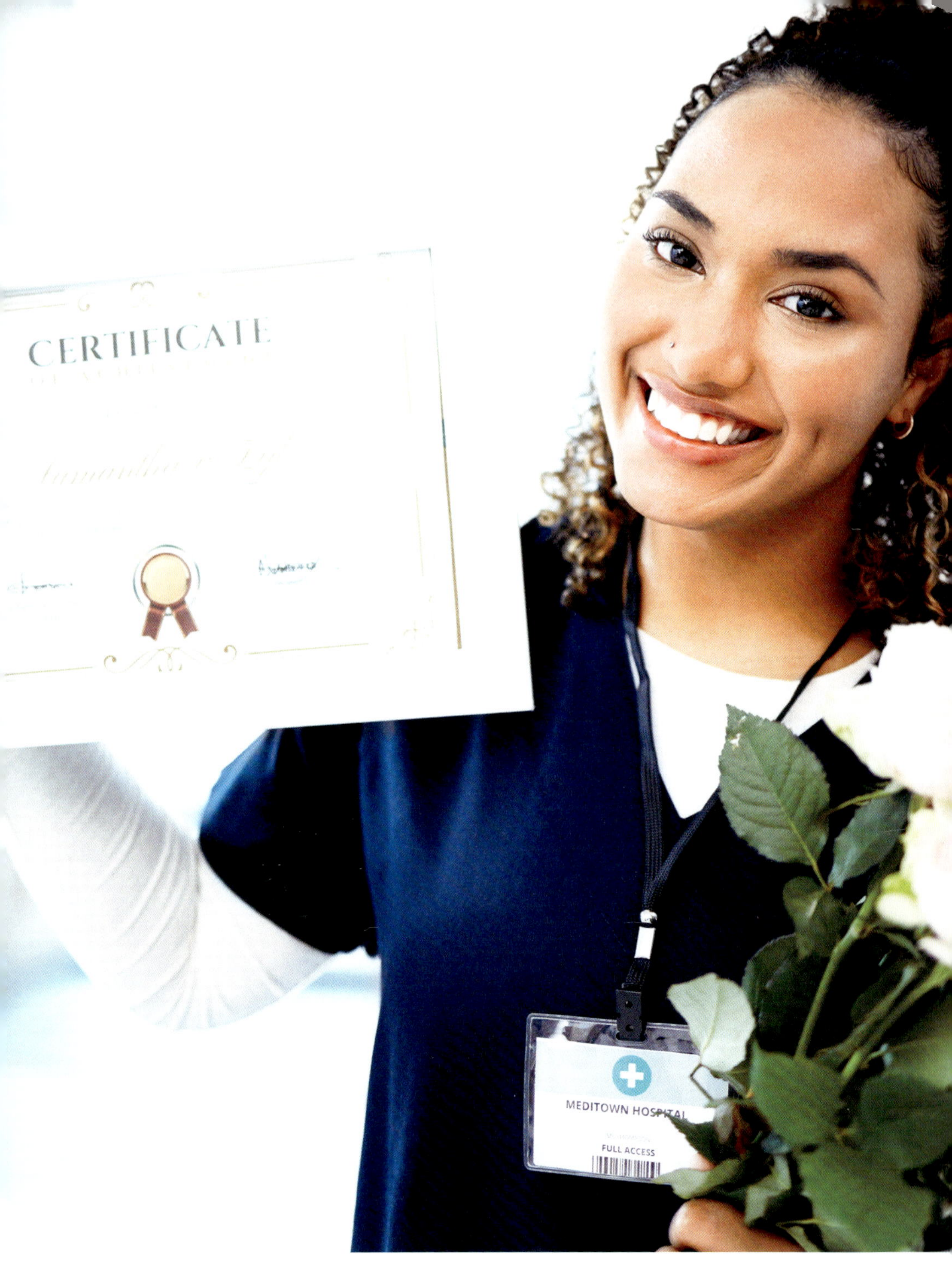

A graduate ceremony is a time for students to celebrate their hard work.

many rewards. An NP gets to work with other passionate health care professionals. They also meet patients of all different backgrounds. Jen Wiles is a family NP. She says,

> *Working as a[n] NP, you get to directly affect lives on a daily basis. You meet needs when someone is at their lowest point. It is a rewarding but challenging role. . . . I never imagined after graduating from a Family NP program that I would be caring for patients with such complex medical conditions. Taking care of these patients from their first day in the hospital to their last revealed the impact you can truly have on a person's health.*[4]

CHAPTER THREE

A DAY IN THE LIFE OF A NURSE PRACTITIONER

An NP's daily routine varies. Hours, workplaces, and job duties depend on specialty. All NPs work on teams. Each team includes medical assistants and doctors. NPs communicate with patients. They keep them up to date on medical care options. Some NPs supervise and train other nurses. They may also record patient information, order supplies, or set schedules.

Some NPs are scheduled for 12-hour shifts. They may work through the day or all night.

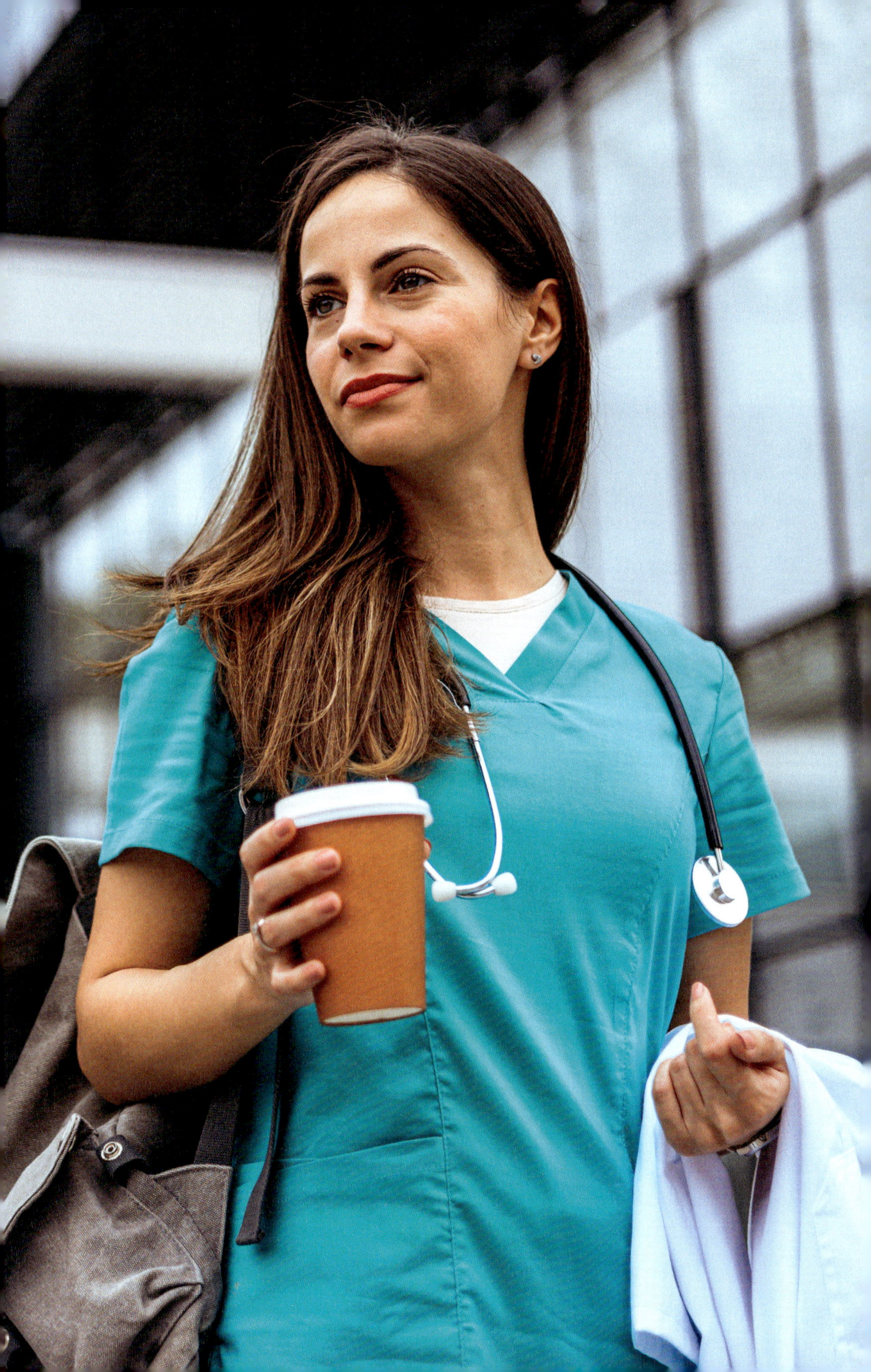

Attention to detail is an important skill for all NPs. Primary care NPs and acute care NPs assess patients. They check blood pressure and heart rate. They look at body weight and lung capacity. They look for lumps on the skin. NPs who work in ERs

In emergencies, ambulances provide safe, fast transport to care facilities so patients can get the care they need.

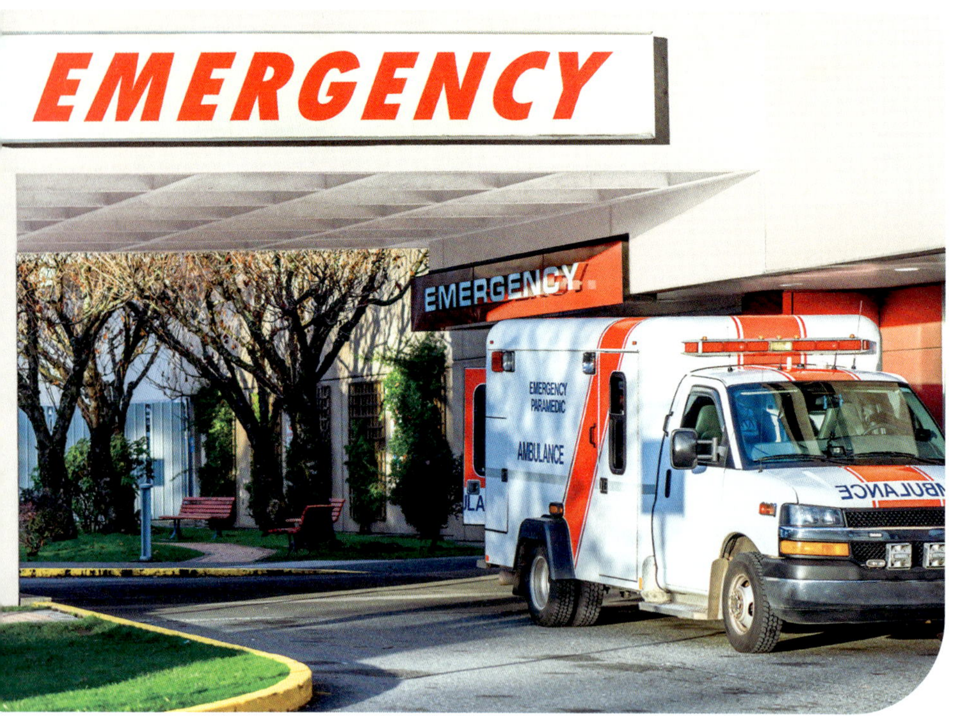

might need to do these tasks more quickly. They need to stay calm. They think through problems under pressure.

A DAY IN THE LIFE OF A PRIMARY CARE NP

Tiffany has been an NP at a health care center in New York City for 10 years. She works in family practice. Tiffany studied biochemistry for her 4-year degree. Later, she became an RN, and then an NP.

Tiffany says, "Being an NP in a major city is amazing. I love working with such a diverse population. There are so many different cultures. And I also get to see a large variety of cases."[5]

Tiffany works from 9:00 a.m. to 5:00 p.m. She sees about twenty patients each day at the health care center. When she gets to work, she goes to her computer. She reads messages from patients and coworkers. She reads lab and test results for her patients.

One of Tiffany's first patients is Maria. She is short of breath. She has asthma. This is a lung disease. It can cause airways to close. This makes it hard for Maria to breathe. Tiffany uses her **stethoscope** and listens to Maria's lungs. She can tell by the sound of Maria's breathing that her airways are tight. Tiffany sets Maria up with a machine. A mask covers Maria's mouth and nose. It sends medicine into Maria's lungs. After the treatment, Maria can breathe more easily. Tiffany prescribes her a steroid inhaler. It will help Marie breathe.

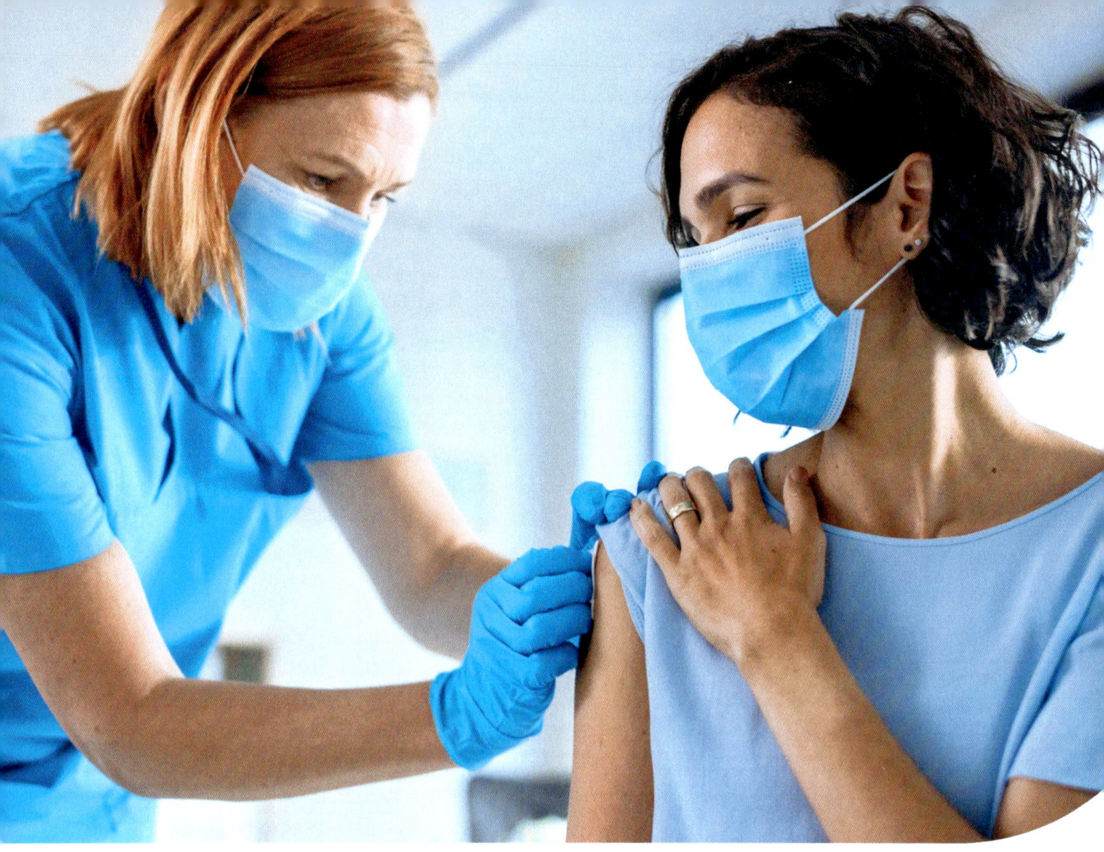

NPs wear medical face masks and gloves when working with patients to protect against germs.

Later that morning, Tiffany sees Aisha. Aisha has a cough and **congestion**. Tiffany listens to Aisha's heart and lungs. She checks her ears, throat, and nose. She does a COVID-19 test. The test is negative.

Aisha most likely has a cold virus. It is making her feel unwell. Tiffany prescribes cough medicine. She tells her to come back if she is not better in a week. Tiffany then takes a 1-hour lunch break.

After Tiffany's break, she sees another patient. Amy is a young woman with chest pain. Tiffany asks Amy to show her where it hurts. Amy holds her right hand to her chest. Tiffany asks more questions. She learns Amy's father has heart disease. This makes it more likely that she might, too. Tiffany listens to her heart. She orders an electrocardiogram (EKG). This test measures the rhythm, strength, and pace of the heart. It can show blocked arteries or poor blood flow. Tiffany sees signs of heart disease on the EKG.

Tiffany gives Amy some aspirin, chest pain medicine, and oxygen. This will help relieve her symptoms. Then Tiffany checks in with a doctor. The doctor agrees that Amy should be taken to the ER for further testing.

A DAY IN THE LIFE OF AN EMERGENCY ROOM NP

James is an NP in the ER of a hospital. His work hours vary. Some weeks he works three 12-hour shifts. Other weeks he works five 8-hour shifts. His shifts can be day or night. They can be weekdays

NP Statistics

NPs who work full-time write an average of twenty-one prescriptions per day. About 57 percent of NPs see at least three patients per hour. The average NP has been in practice for 9 years. The average age of an NP is 46 years old.

or weekends. Sometimes James works on holidays.

Today, James's work shift is from 6:00 p.m. to 2:00 a.m. He must get a lot of rest. When most people are finishing their workday, James is about to start his. He sees about twenty patients per 8-hour shift

Night shifts for NPs can be tiring, as fewer medical staff members are working.

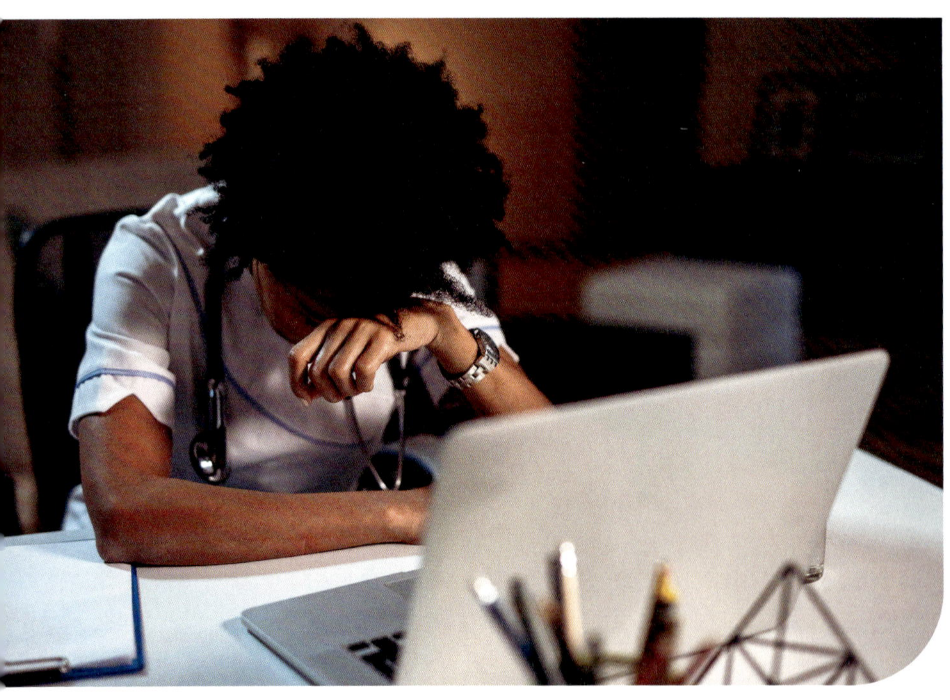

at the hospital. When James arrives, there are many patients. The ER is always busy.

James's first patient has stomach pain. He examines him. He suspects the man has kidney stones. Kidney stones are made up of solid minerals and salts. They may cause pain when moving through the kidneys or bladder. James has seen these symptoms many times before. He orders some pain medicine for the patient. He orders a test and some lab work to confirm the diagnosis.

James's next patient has been in a car accident. Her wrist hurts. She has a splint on her wrist. James removes it carefully. The wrist is swollen and bruised. He orders pain medicine and an X-ray. It will tell him if the wrist bone is broken.

Another patient was doing some home repairs. He accidentally hammered a nail into his finger. James orders an X-ray. The nail is stuck far into the bone. James tries to pull it out. But it is painful for the patient. James calls in a doctor to help. Together they remove the nail. James then prescribes **antibiotics** to prevent infection. He also updates the patient's medical record. James provides instructions to the patient to return to the hospital if he experiences any feelings of pain or sickness. After James's long shift, he goes home and rests.

James enjoys working in the ER. He likes the fast-paced work. He says, "In the ER, I never know what each day will bring. I see patients with chest pain, abdominal pain, joint, and bone problems. I do procedures

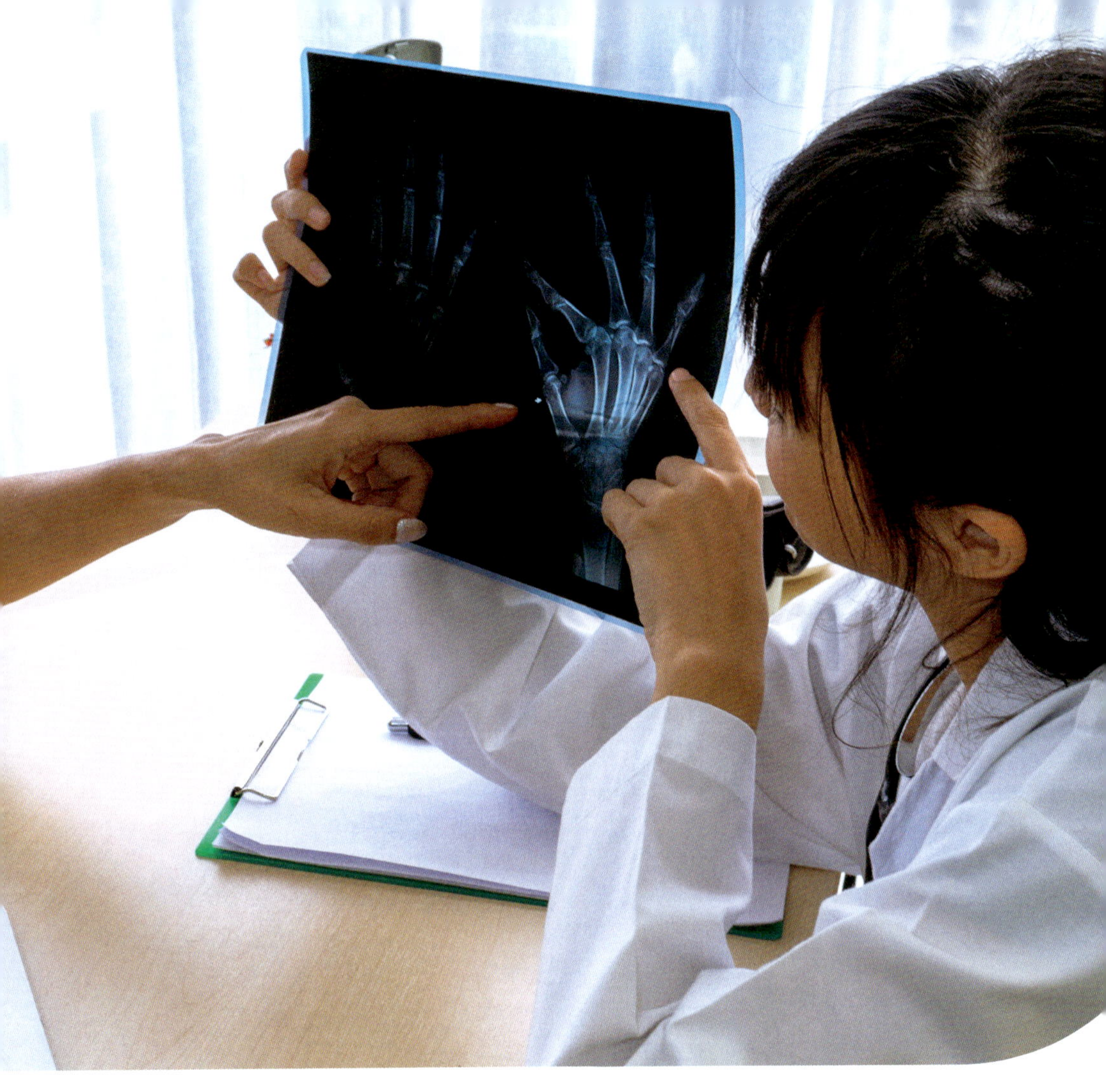

X-rays and other scans can help NPs diagnose broken bones and other issues.

such as drain pus and close wounds. I enjoy the variety and challenges my job provides. I learn new things every day. I love my job and highly recommend the nurse practitioner career."[6]

CHAPTER FOUR

THE OUTLOOK FOR NURSE PRACTITIONERS

There are many reasons for choosing a career as an NP. The outlook for NPs in the United States is strong. The US Bureau of Labor Statistics (BLS) is a federal agency. It collects, analyzes, and posts data on the US economy. The BLS predicts more than a 40 percent job growth for NPs from 2023 to 2033. This is much faster than the average of 4 percent growth for other jobs. NPs make a competitive salary as well. In 2024,

NPs socialize with patients and other medical staff every day.

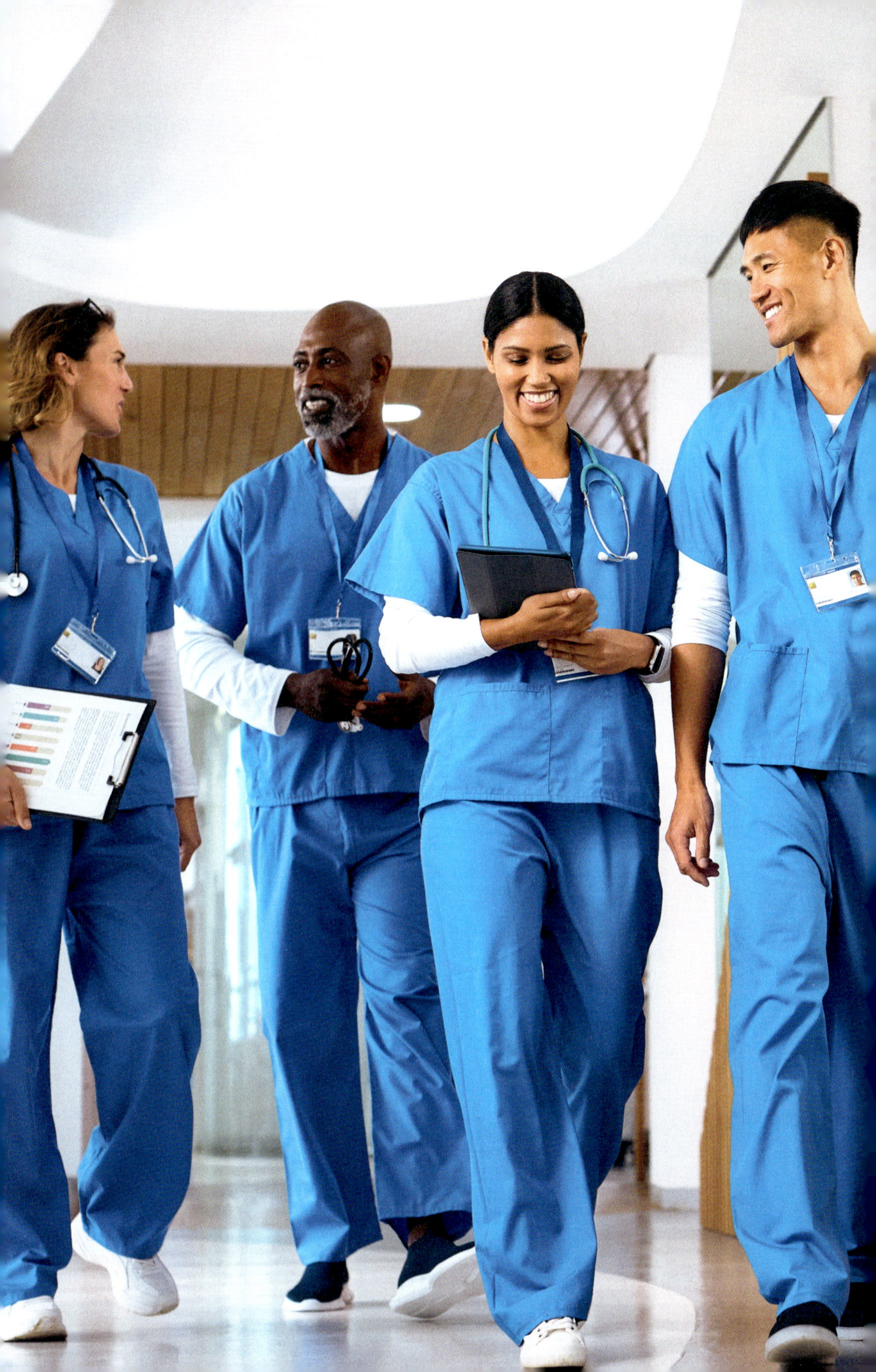

their average earnings were $128,000. This is about twice as much as the US average earnings for all jobs.

In the United States, there is a growing shortage of primary care providers. More states are granting full practice authority

NPs play important roles in keeping communities strong and healthy.

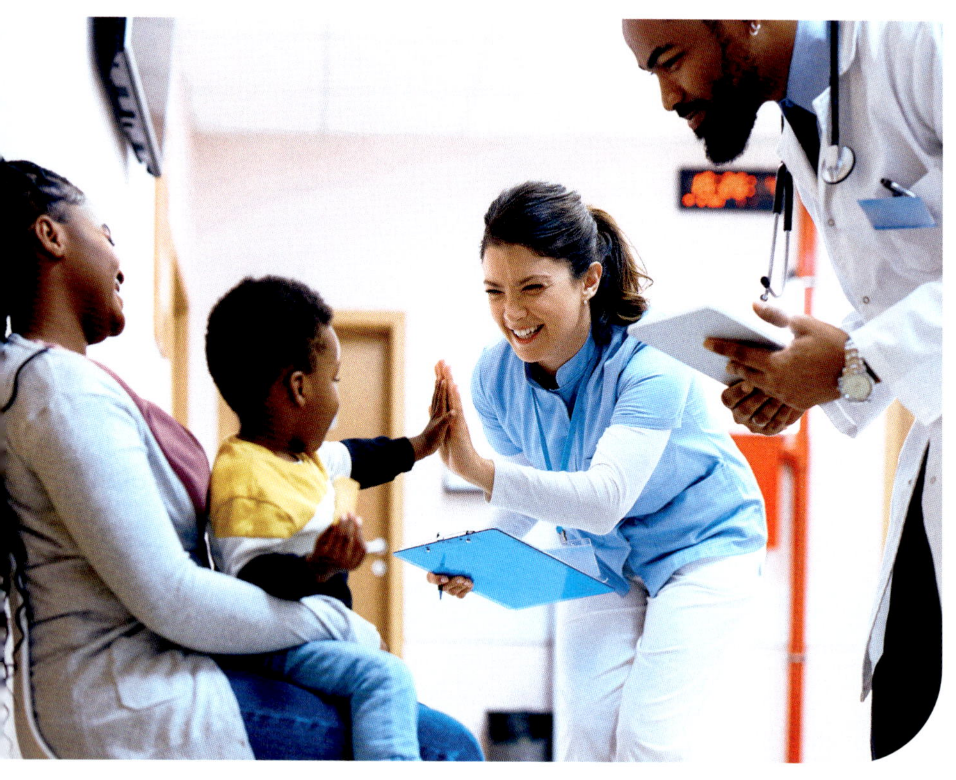

to NPs. This means they can do most of the tasks that doctors do.

A GROWING SHORTAGE

The American Association of Medical Colleges (AAMC) predicts that by 2034, there will be a shortage of doctors in the United States. They say 37,800 to 124,000 doctors will be needed to fill jobs. In the next decade, more than 40 percent of doctors will likely retire. At the same time, the number of seniors will increase. Seniors tend to need more primary care. They need wellness tests and checks. Seniors are also more likely to have chronic illnesses that require consistent treatment.

Clinics can hire primary care NPs to fill doctor shortages. In full practice authority states, NPs prescribe, diagnose, and treat patients. They can do this without doctor supervision. NPs can open and run their own clinics. In reduced authority states, NPs can diagnose and treat patients. But they need doctor supervision to prescribe medicine. In restricted authority states, NPs need doctor supervision for most tasks.

NPs in doctor's offices may help lower the cost of health care by one-third. Patient visits with NPs are usually less costly than with doctors. This is especially true in full practice authority states. An education advisor for *Forbes* magazine writes, "Patients who see NPs as their primary health care providers tend to have lower medication costs, shorter hospital stays, and fewer visits to the ER."[7]

AVERAGE SALARY FOR NURSE PRACTITIONERS BY SPECIALTY

Nurse Practitioner Specialties	Salary Ranges
Family Nurse Practitioner	$106,382–$138,328
Acute Care Nurse Practitioner	$111,242–$131,201
Pediatric Nurse Practitioner	$98,787–$127,948
Emergency Room Nurse Practitioner	$99,044–$134,720
Neonatal Nurse Practitioner	$114,259–$137,460
Psychiatric Mental Health Nurse Practitioner	$118,710–$127,041
Women's Health Nurse Practitioner	$101,186–$133,810
Gerontology Primary Care Nurse Practitioner	$106,566–$117,532

Source: "Nurse Practitioner Salary–By Specialty & State," Nurse Practitioner Online, *February 13, 2024. www.nursepractitioneronline.com.*

There are many NP specialties. This chart shows the median salaries earned by different NP specialties in 2024 according to popular salary reporting websites.

FUTURE JOB TRENDS

Home health care is becoming more popular. It helps people get medical care without leaving their homes. For patients who are sick or hurt, getting to a clinic might be hard. Home visits from NPs can help. Telehealth services are also on the rise. These services allow NPs to provide care from a distance. It might be with a phone or video call. In areas without nearby clinics, patients can still get medical help.

Traveling NPs work in different locations across the country. They are usually assigned work in areas that have a shortage of health care professionals. They may work

Diversity in the NP Workforce

In 2021, more than 85 percent of NPs were women and 75 percent were white. In 2023, nearly 12 percent of all LNs, RNs, and NPs were men. A more diverse NP team allows for more personalized care. It means having a diversity of gender, racial, and cultural identities to support patients with different backgrounds.

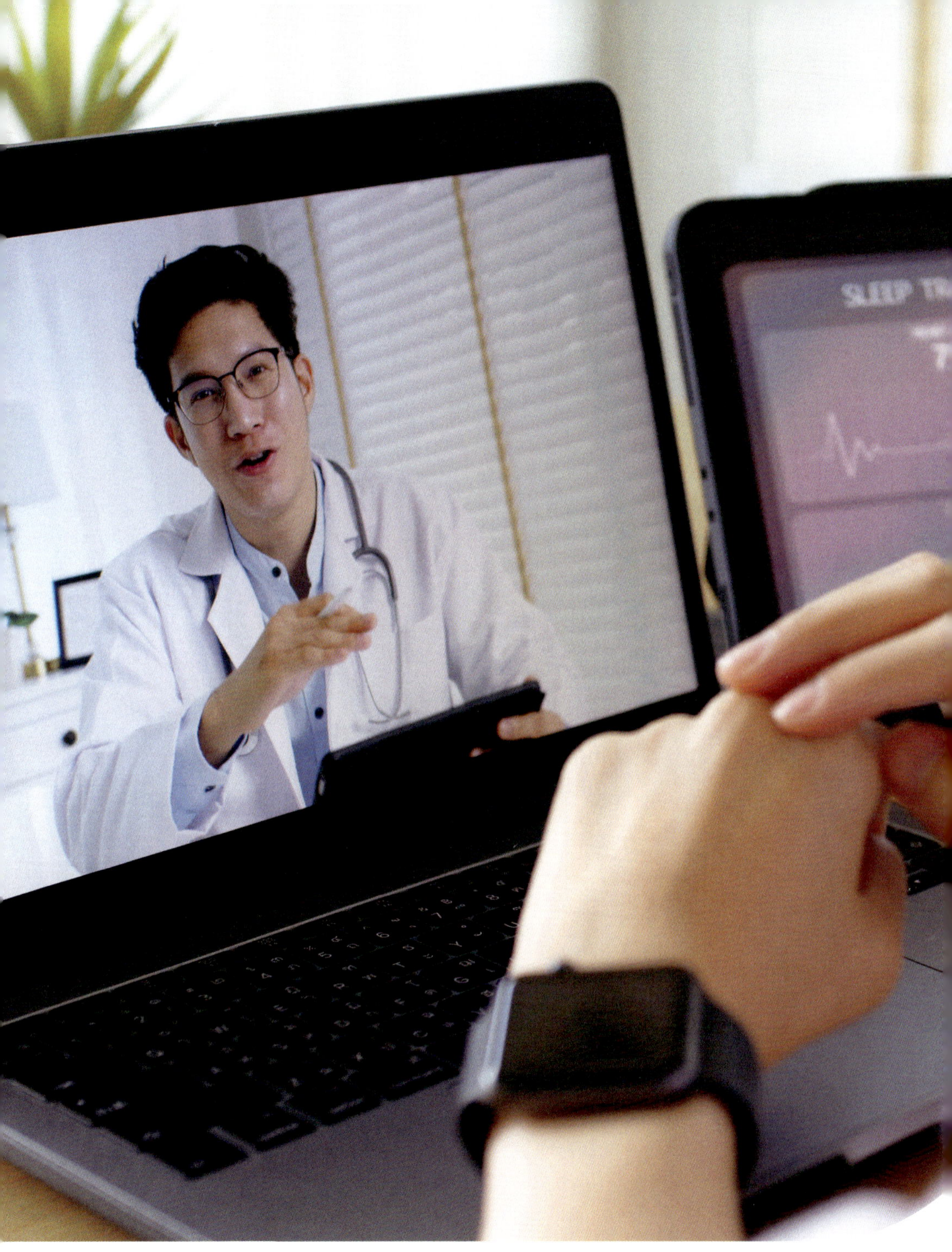

A stable internet connection is needed to use telehealth services.

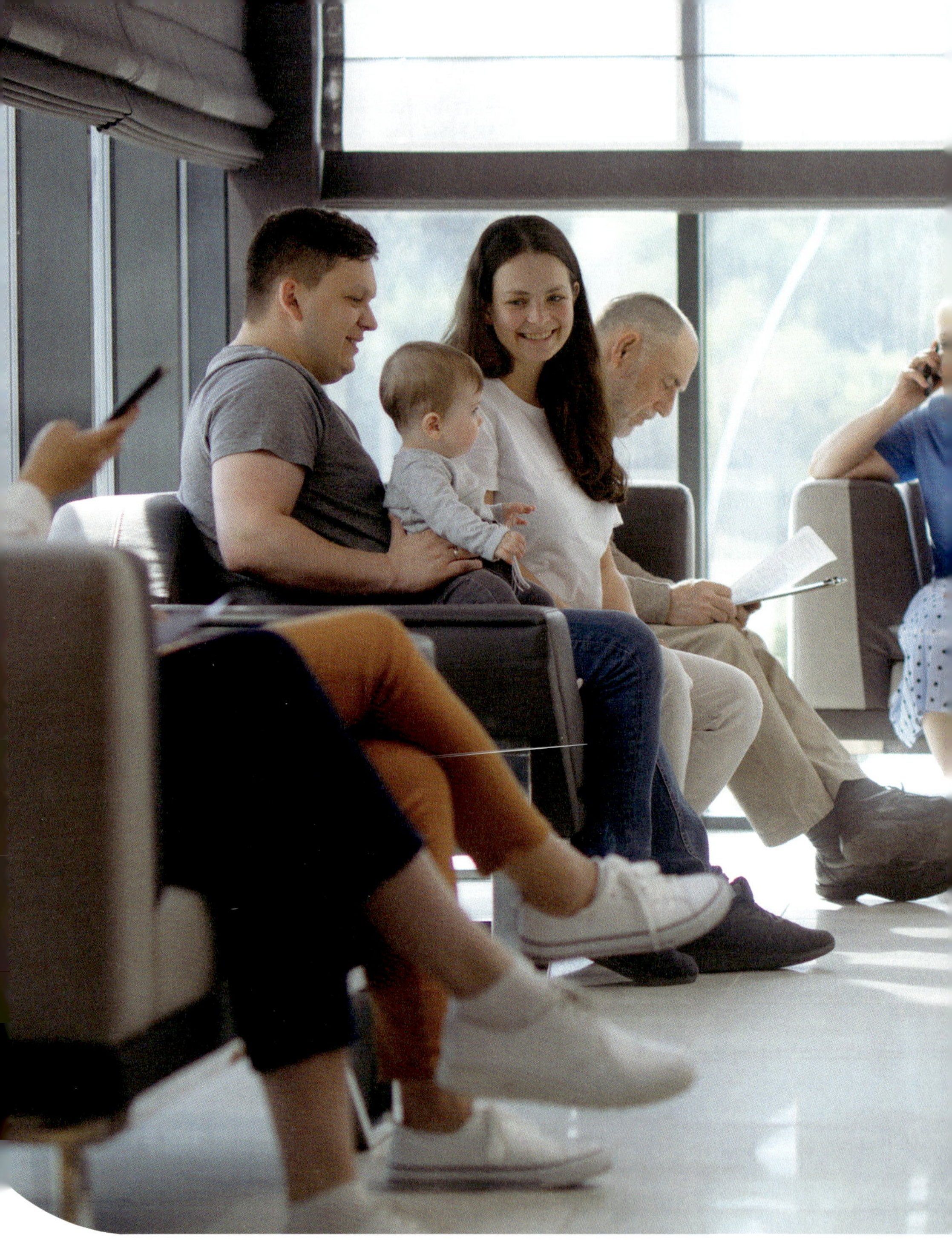

Being able to connect with patients of all ages is important for primary care NPs.

anywhere from 2 weeks to 26 weeks. These NPs are provided with housing money and travel allowances. This helps them focus on providing care to patients.

A career as an NP offers many advantages. NPs have a wide range of choices. They have many types of specialties to choose from. NPs also work in different places. They may also set their own schedules. Their skills are in high demand. The work is also rewarding. Erin Tolbert is an NP. She says, "I love working as a nurse practitioner. My job is interesting, challenging, and fun. I work hard, but I enjoy my flexible schedule. I highly recommend a career as a nurse practitioner to anyone interested in health care."[8]

GLOSSARY

allergen

a substance that causes an allergic reaction

antibiotics

medicine that kills microorganisms that cause illness

chronic conditions

illnesses that last for long periods of time

congestion

the build-up of something, such as mucus in the nose or lungs

diabetes

a disease in which the body does not make or process insulin, causing high blood sugar

diagnoses

identifies a disease by examining or testing a patient

reproductive health care

health care that relates to the physical, mental, and social well-being of someone's reproductive systems

stethoscope

a medical tool used to listen to a patient's heart and lungs

transfusions

putting blood from a donor into a person's circulatory system

SOURCE NOTES

INTRODUCTION: UNSUNG HERO

1. Quoted in Autumn Barnes, "No One Could Figure Out the Cause of Her Cough. Then a Nurse Practitioner Had an Idea," *National Public Radio*, February 21, 2024. www.npr.org.

CHAPTER ONE: WHAT DOES A NURSE PRACTITIONER DO?

2. Quoted in "What Is Primary Care?" *UC Davis Health*, June 29, 2023. https://health.ucdavis.edu.

3. Quoted in "Acute Care vs. Primary Care NPs: How Are They Different?" *University of Tulsa*, August 3, 2023. https://online.utulsa.edu.

CHAPTER TWO: BECOMING A NURSE PRACTITIONER

4. Quoted in Kaitlin Louie, "Interview with Jen Wiles, FNP-BC," *Online FNP Programs*, 2023. www.onlinefnpprograms.com.

CHAPTER THREE: A DAY IN THE LIFE OF A NURSE PRACTITIONER

5. Quoted in "What Is a Day in the Life of a Nurse Practitioner Like?" *Indeed*, July 30, 2024. https://www.indeed.com.

6. Quoted in, "A Day in the Life of an ER Nurse Practitioner," *ThriveAP*, n.d. https://provider.thriveap.com.

CHAPTER FOUR: THE OUTLOOK FOR NURSE PRACTITIONERS

7. Quoted in Nneoma Uche, "How to Become A Nurse Practitioner: A Step-By-Step Guide," *Forbes*, January 4, 2024. www.forbes.com.

8. Quoted in Erin Tolbert, "What's a Day in the Life of a Nurse Practitioner Really Like?" *Health eCareers*, May 29, 2019. www.healthecareers.com.

FOR FURTHER RESEARCH

BOOKS

Mike Downs, *Become a Respiratory Therapist.* BrightPoint Press, 2025.

Cathleen Small, *How to Choose Your Perfect Healthcare Career.* Cheriton Children's Books, 2023.

Marne Ventura, *Become a Licensed Practical Nurse.* BrightPoint Press, 2025.

INTERNET SOURCES

Allie Blackham, "How To Become a Nurse Practitioner in 7 Steps (Plus FAQs)," *Indeed*, December 30, 2024. www.indeed.com.

"How to Become a Nurse Practitioner: A Practical Guide," *University of St. Augustine for Health Sciences*, September 18, 2024. www.usa.edu.

"What is a Nurse Practitioner?" *American Nurses Association Hub*, February 9, 2024. www.nursingworld.org.

WEBSITES

American Association of Nurse Practitioners

www.aanp.org

The American Association of Nurse Practitioners website presents an overview of the NP career. It explains different workplaces, specialties, and benefits.

Lippincott Nursing Center

www.nursingcenter.com

The Lippincott Nursing Center is an online source for nursing journals. There are free newsletters with nursing news and patient educational materials.

Mayo Clinic College of Medicine and Science

https://college.mayo.edu

The Mayo Clinic College of Medicine and Science website provides a list of health care roles. It also has information on steps to become an NP.

INDEX

IMAGE CREDITS

Cover: © Meeko Media/Shutterstock Images
5: © Pixel-Shot/Shutterstock Images
7: © Jacob Lund/Shutterstock Images
8: © Art_Photo/Shutterstock Images
10: © Ground Picture/Shutterstock Images
11: © antoniodiaz/Shutterstock Images
12: © Gorodenkoff/Shutterstock Images
15: © PeopleImages.com-Yuri A./Shutterstock Images
17: © Westock Productions/Shutterstock Images
19: © Halfpoint/Shutterstock Images
22: © Oksana Sahinoglu/Shutterstock Images
25: © Pixel-Shot/Shutterstock Images
26: © PeopleImages.com-Yuri A./Shutterstock Images
29: © ESB Professional/Shutterstock Images
31: © Africa Studio/Shutterstock Images
33: © Bongkarn Graphic/Shutterstock Images
34: © PeopleImages.com-Yuri A./Shutterstock Images
37: © Dragana Gordic/Shutterstock Images
38: © Viktor Birkus/Shutterstock Images
41: © Gorodenkoff/Shutterstock Images
44: © Drazen Zigic/Shutterstock Images
47: © katobonsai/Shutterstock Images
49: © Monkey Business Images/Shutterstock Images
50: © Drazen Zigic/Shutterstock Images
53: © Red Line Editorial
55: © Chay_Tee/Shutterstock Images
56: © Frame Stock Footage/Shutterstock Images

ABOUT THE AUTHOR

Marne Ventura is the author of more than 150 books for young people. A former elementary school teacher, she holds a master's degree in reading and language development from the University of California. Ventura's nonfiction titles cover a wide range of topics, including careers, media literacy, STEM, and biographies. Ventura and her family live in California.